ANGELA RAMOS

Curly Hair Hacks

Understanding and Managing Your Waves, Coils, and Curls

This book was professionally typeset on Reedsy.
Find out more at reedsy.com

Contents

1

Chapter 1:Embrace Your Curly Crown

D o you remember when curly hair felt like a secret struggle? Back in the 80s, being a curly-haired Latina meant dealing with the daily chorus of "kinky hair" and "bad hair." Our hair was misunderstood, and as for products? Let's say it was a wild west of hair care. Remember Dep and LA Looks? If those names sound like relics from a distant past, count yourself lucky. You've grown up in an era where products are formulated with love and care and smell like flowers and honey, not some mysterious concoction of chemicals.

But here's the thing: Even in today's curl-friendly world, managing curly hair can sometimes feel like an uphill battle. It's like having a rebellious best friend who doesn't always want to play by the rules. Yet, we wouldn't have it any other way.

So, why this book? It's here to be your trusty guide on your journey to healthier, happier hair. Flip through the pages, dive into the table of contents, and discover an arsenal of curly hair hacks to breathe life back into those gorgeous waves, curls, and coils. Your hair is more than just a bunch of strands; it's an extension of your personality, beauty, and confidence. We want it to look its absolute best, but let's be honest, sometimes it has a mind of its own.

I'm not a professional hairstylist but a professional curly girl who cares about others like me. I understand the frustration of staring into the mirror and wondering why your hair won't cooperate. And that's why I'm here—because you deserve to love your curls daily.

So, whether you're a seasoned curl connoisseur or just starting your journey, this book is for you. Let's unravel the mysteries of curly hair together, discover tips and tricks, and unlock the secrets to having your best hair day every day. It's time to embrace your curly crown and let your unique beauty shine!

1.1 Understanding the Types of Curls

Curls come in all shapes and sizes, just like people! Whether you're trying to style your hair or just curious about the different curl types, this guide will help you understand the basics without getting too tangled up in technical jargon.

1. Straight Hair: Let's start with the basics. Straight hair is naturally sleek and has no noticeable curls or waves. It's smooth and can be pretty easy to manage.
2. Wavy Hair: If your hair has gentle, subtle waves that resemble soft "S" shapes, you likely have wavy hair. This type of hair is not too curly but not entirely straight.
3. Curly Hair: When your hair forms well-defined, round curls, These curls can range from loose to tight, adding a lot of texture and volume to your hair.

4. Coily or Kinky Hair: Coily hair has tight, small curls that often resemble a zigzag pattern. It's also known as kinky or afro-textured hair. Coily hair can be very thick and needs extra care to keep it moisturized.

Now, let's dive deeper into the subcategories of curly hair:

1. Loose Curls (Type 2): If you have gentle, flowing curls that aren't too tight, you fall into the Type 2 category. It can range from barely noticeable waves (2A) to more defined and pronounced waves (2B and 2C). These curls often look like beach waves and are pretty manageable.
2. Tight Curls (Type 3): Type 3 curls are more defined and springy. They can range from loose curls to corkscrew curls. These curls can vary from loose and bouncy (3A) to more tightly coiled (3B) or even springy corkscrew curls (3C). This hair type benefits from regular hydration and specialized styling products.
3. Very Tight Curls (Type 4): Type 4 curls are the tightest. They can appear as coils or zigzags, and this hair type can be pretty delicate.

It is further subdivided into Type 4A, 4B, and 4C, with 4A having more defined curls, 4B forming a tighter coil, and 4C having a zigzag pattern with minimal curl definition. Coily hair is typically very dense and can shrink significantly when dry. Keeping it moisturized and protected is crucial.

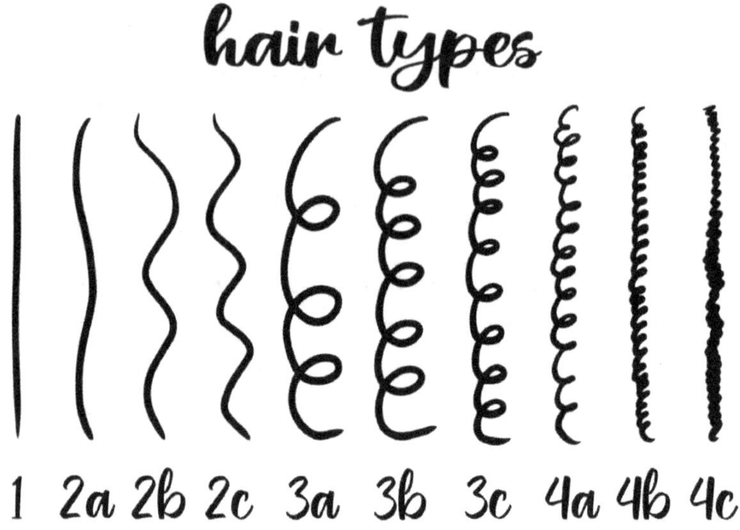

These curl types are just general guidelines, and many people have different curl patterns on their heads. Additionally, it's important to note that hair texture can vary widely within each curl type, from fine to coarse and from high porosity (absorbs moisture quickly) to low porosity (resists moisture absorption).

Understanding your curl type and texture can help you choose the right hair care products and styling techniques to maintain healthy and beautiful curls. Remember that everyone's hair is unique, so what works best for one person may not work for another, and embracing your natural curls is always a great choice!

1.2 The Science Behind Curly Hair

Have you ever wondered why some people have straight hair while others have those beautiful curls? Well, it all comes down to science, and today, we're going to unravel the mysteries behind those curly locks in a way that even a teenager or an adult can understand.

1. Hair Shape:

The shape of your hair follicles plays a crucial role. Imagine your hair follicles as tiny tunnels in your scalp where each hair strand grows. You're more likely to have straight hair if these tunnels are round. But you'll have curly hair if they're more oval or twisted.

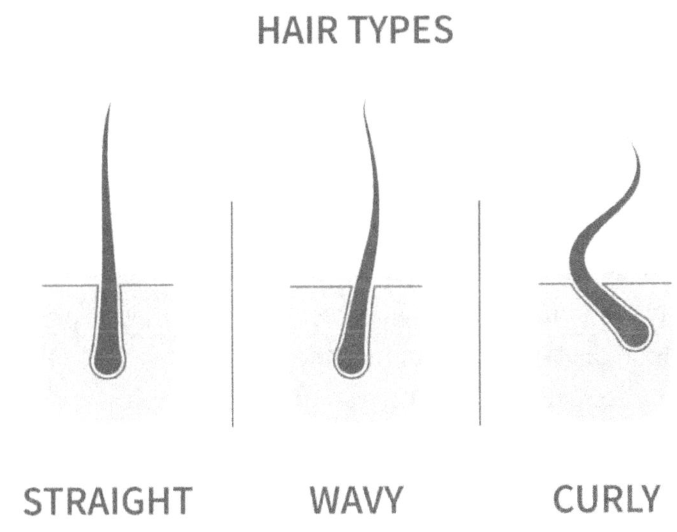

2. Hair Protein:

Now, let's talk about the stuff that makes up your hair: keratin protein. This protein forms the structure of your hair strands. Straight hair has a more uniform distribution of keratin, making it smooth and refined. But the keratin isn't evenly spread out in curly hair, causing twists and turns we love so much.

3. Bonds Between Atoms:

The bonds between atoms in its protein structure influence your hair's shape. These bonds have three types: hydrogen, salt, and disulfide.

- Hydrogen Bonds: These are like temporary ties between atoms in your hair and form when your hair gets wet. As your hair dries, these bonds can cause it to change from straight to curly or vice versa temporarily.
- Salt Bonds: Like hydrogen bonds, salt bonds are temporary and can change your hair's shape when wet. However, they also return to their original shape as your hair dries.
- Disulfide Bonds: These are the strongest and most essential bonds for your hair's permanent shape. The number of disulfide bonds in your hair determines whether it's straight or curly. More disulfide bonds mean curlier hair.

4. Genetics:

Genes from your parents play a huge role in your hair type. If your mom or dad has curly hair, you're more likely to have it too. It's like passing down a curly hair instruction manual in your DNA!

5. Environmental Factors:

Your hair can also change over time due to humidity. Curly hair tends to absorb moisture from the air, causing it to swell and get curlier. Conversely, dry conditions can make it lose some of its curl.

So, in a nutshell, the science of curly hair boils down to the shape of your hair follicles, the distribution of keratin, the types of bonds in your hair, your genetics, and environmental factors. It's a fascinating mix of biology and chemistry, giving us unique and beautiful curls. Embrace your natural hair type and rock those curls with confidence!

2

Chapter 2: Basic Care and Maintenance

2.1 Proper Shampooing Techniques for Curly Hair Types

Keeping those gorgeous curls looking their best can be tricky. Correctly Shampooing your curls is a crucial step in your hair care routine. Let's break down some easy-to-follow steps for proper curly hair shampooing, and we'll also discuss where you can find information about the ingredients in your hair products.

1. Choose the Right Shampoo:

- Look for a sulfate-free shampoo. Sulfates can be harsh on curly hair and strip away natural oils, leading to dryness and frizz.
- Check for shampoos labeled as "hydrating," "moisturizing," or "curl-enhancing." These are designed to add moisture to your curls.

2. Wet Your Hair Thoroughly:

- Before applying shampoo, make sure your hair is completely wet. It helps the shampoo distribute evenly.

3. Use a Small Amount of Shampoo:

- Less is more when it comes to shampooing curly hair. You don't need a lot of products. Start with a quarter-sized amount and adjust as needed.

4. Focus on the scalp:

- Gently massage the shampoo into your scalp with your fingertips. Don't rub vigorously, as this can tangle your curls.

5. Let the Shampoo Run Down:

- As you rinse the shampoo from your scalp, let it naturally run down the length of your hair. It helps cleanse your curls without over-drying them.

6. Conditioner is Your Friend:

- After shampooing, use a conditioner that matches your hair type. Apply it mainly to the mid-lengths and ends of your hair, where curls are drier.
- Detangle your hair with a wide-toothed comb or your fingers while the conditioner is in. It will help prevent breakage.

7. Rinse Thoroughly:

- Rinse out the conditioner thoroughly. Leaving some in can make your hair feel greasy.

8. Use a Microfiber Towel or T-shirt:

- Avoid rough drying with a regular towel, as it can cause frizz. Instead, gently squeeze excess water from your hair using a microfiber towel or an old t-shirt.

9. Avoid Heat:

- Let your hair air dry, or use a diffuser attachment on your hairdryer if needed. Avoid high heat settings to prevent damage.

10. Product Ingredient Information:

- You can check the product labels to determine what ingredients are in your hair products. Most products list their ingredients on the packaging.
- You can also visit the manufacturer's website or contact customer service for ingredient information if it's not listed on the packaging.

Finding the right shampoo and conditioner for your curly hair type might take some experimentation. Everyone's curls are unique, so don't be discouraged if it takes a bit of trial and error to discover the best products for you. With proper shampooing and care, you can keep your curls looking fabulous!

2.2 The Importance of Deep Conditioning for Curly Hair

Deep conditioning is a crucial step in caring for curly hair. Let's explain why it's so important and provide information on where you can find ingredient details in hair products.

Deep conditioning is like giving your curls a big drink of water and a warm hug. Here's why it's essential for curly hair:

1. Hydration: Curly hair tends to be drier because natural oils have difficulty traveling down the spiral-shaped strands. Deep conditioning adds much-needed moisture, making your curls softer, smoother, and more manageable.

2. Reduces Frizz: Dry hair often leads to frizz. Deep conditioning helps seal the hair's cuticles. These are like tiny protective layers on each strand. When the cuticles lay flat, your hair is less likely to frizz.

3. Improves Elasticity: Healthy curls have good bounce and stretch. Deep conditioning can enhance your hair's elasticity, making it less prone to breakage.

4. Repairs Damage: If your curls are damaged from heat styling or chemical treatments, deep conditioning can help repair and restore them, making your hair look and feel healthier.

5. Enhances Curl Definition: Proper deep conditioning can make your curls more defined and pop with vibrancy.

Now, let's talk about how you can find out what ingredients are in your hair products:

Apps and Websites for Checking Hair Product Ingredients:

Think Dirty: This app allows you to scan or search for personal care products, including hair conditioners and provides information on potentially harmful ingredients.

CosDNA: CosDNA is a website where you can look up ingredients in skincare and haircare products. It provides detailed information on the safety and potential irritants of each ingredient.

EWG's Skin Deep: The Environmental Working Group's Skin Deep database rates the safety of personal care products and their ingredients. You can search for your hair conditioner to see its safety rating.

Curlsbot: Curlsbot is a website specifically designed for those with curly hair. It helps you identify curly girl method-approved products by analyzing ingredients.

InciDecoder: InciDecoder is a website that explains skincare and haircare ingredients in plain language. You can search for products or ingredients to learn more about their properties.

Ingredients to Look for in Curly Hair Conditioners:

Shea Butter: Shea butter is rich in moisture-locking fatty acids and can deeply hydrate and nourish curly hair.

Coconut Oil: Coconut oil helps reduce protein loss in hair, making it stronger and less prone to breakage. It also adds moisture and shine.

Glycerin: Glycerin is a humectant that attracts and retains moisture, helping to keep your curls hydrated.

Aloe Vera: Aloe vera has soothing and hydrating properties that can calm frizz and promote healthy hair growth.

Jojoba Oil: Jojoba oil is similar to the natural oils produced by your scalp, making it an excellent conditioner and moisturizer for curly hair.

When looking at conditioner ingredients, paying attention to what your hair needs explicitly is essential. Curly hair can vary in texture and porosity, so different ingredients work better for your unique curls. Always check for allergens or ingredients that may not agree with your hair type.

When you're looking at the ingredient list, keep an eye out for things like sulfates (which can be drying for curls), silicones (which can cause buildup), and alcohol (which can be drying). Look for nourishing ingredients like natural oils, shea butter, and glycerin, which can benefit curly hair.

In summary, deep conditioning is crucial for maintaining healthy, beautiful curls by providing essential moisture and protection. To find out what ingredients are in your hair products, check the product labels, visit the manufacturer's website, contact customer service, or use online resources and apps dedicated to ingredient information. Your curly hair can look and feel best with proper care and attention!

2.3 The Importance of Regular Trimming for Curly Hair

Imagine your curls as a beautiful garden. To keep that garden looking lush and healthy, you need to do a bit of pruning now and then. Here's why regular trimming is like tending to your curly hair garden:

1. Prevents Split Ends:

Curly hair can develop split ends like a garden can get overgrown and messy. These are like little splits or breaks in your hair strands. Trimming removes them, preventing them from traveling up the hair shaft and causing more damage.

2. Promotes Healthy Growth:

When you trim your hair regularly, you're getting rid of the oldest and often most damaged parts; this makes room for new, healthier hair to grow. It's like weeding your garden to make space for fresh, vibrant flowers.

3. Enhances Curl Definition:

Trimming helps your curls bounce back and spring into action. When the ends are tidy and free from damage, your rings tend to look more defined and lively.

4. Reduces frizz:

Over time, the tips of your curls can get rough and contribute to frizz. Trimming those rough ends smoothens your curls, reducing frizz and making your hair look sleeker.

5. Maintains Shape and Style:

If you have a specific curly hairstyle, like layers or bangs, regular trims help maintain the shape and style you love. It's like giving your garden an edge to keep it looking the way you want.

6. Prevents breakage:

When curly hair gets too long without trims, it can become more prone to breakage, especially if it gets tangled. Trimming minimizes the risk of breakage, helping your curls stay strong.

7. Overall Health and Vitality:

Think of regular trims as a way to keep your curly hair garden thriving and flourishing. It's essential to your hair care routine to ensure your curls look their best.

So, remember, just as a well-tended garden grows beautiful flowers, regular trimming helps your curls stay healthy, defined, and full of life. It's a simple but essential step in your curly hair care routine that ensures your locks continue to shine and thrive!

3

Chapter 3: Styling Hacks

3.1 Diffusing vs. Air Drying: Benefits of Each

Diffusing (Using a Hair Dryer with Diffuser Attachment):

1. Faster Drying: Diffusing speeds up the drying process, making it ideal for those in a hurry.
2. Enhanced Volume: It can add volume and bounce to your curls, giving them a more defined look.
3. Reduced Frizz: When used with a low heat and airflow setting, diffusing can help minimize frizz by evenly distributing Heat.
4. Control Over Curls: You can shape and style your curls as you diffuse, achieving a more controlled and uniform result.

Air Drying:

1. Gentle on Hair: Air drying is the gentlest way to dry your curls, reducing the risk of heat damage.
2. Natural Look: It allows your curls to dry naturally, showcasing their

authentic texture and shape.

3. Moisture Retention: Air drying helps retain moisture in your hair, keeping it hydrated and less prone to frizz.
4. Low Maintenance: It's a hassle-free method – just let your hair air dry without needing special equipment.

3.2 Using Silk or Satin Accessories for Frizz-Free Sleep:

1. Sleeping on a silk or satin pillowcase and using silk/satin hair accessories (like scrunchies) can work wonders for curly hair:
2. Reduced Frizz: Silk and satin fabrics create less friction than cotton, preventing frizz and minimizing breakage.
3. Hair Health: They help maintain the natural moisture in your hair, keeping it hydrated and healthy.
4. Preservation of Hairstyles: Silk/satin accessories and pillowcases help preserve your curly hairstyle, so you wake up with less need for restyling.
5. Less Tangling: Curly hair is less likely to tangle on a smooth surface, so silk or satin can help prevent knots.

3.3 DIY Hair Masks for Curly Hair:

Egg Mask for Damaged and Brittle Hair:

If you've been putting a lot of moisture in your hair and it's still dry or damaged, you could need a protein treatment that helps to restore strength. This DIY egg hair mask combines protein-rich eggs, coconut oil, avocado, and hydrating aloe vera and olive oil to enhance suppleness.

Ingredients:
  1-2 eggs
  2 tbsp extra virgin olive oil
  ½ avocado, pitted and chopped
  avocado oil (two teaspoons) (optional)
  1 tbsp coconut oil (optional)
  Spray Bottle

Directions:
  1) Blend all ingredients until completely smooth (no clumps, no

chunks).

2) Section your damaged hair and clip additional sections up and out of the way.

3) Fill a spray bottle halfway with water and moisten each part before applying the mask.

4) Scoop up a little amount of the mask and smooth it through your hair until it's completely soaked, then clip it up and proceed to the next section. If you're working with type-4 hair, skip the clip and instead untangle your hair before braiding it down.

5) Allow at least 20 minutes for your hair to dry after covering it with a shower cap or a grocery bag.

6) Shampoo and condition as usual.

Yogurt Hair Mask to Reduce Breakage and Increase Hair Growth

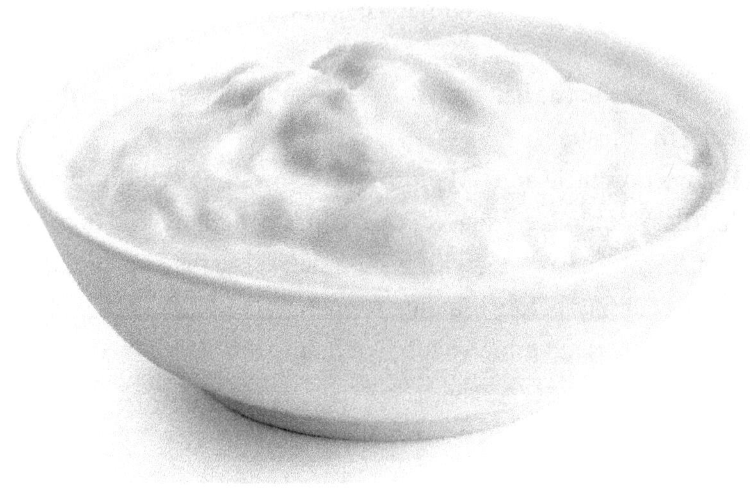

When hair is delicate, dry, and brittle, it breaks – or gets split ends. It can be due to poor styling decisions, but it can also indicate that something is wrong with your diet, and breakage is a warning that you need to increase your protein consumption.

A DIY hair mask made with Greek yogurt, apple cider vinegar, and honey can help your hair repair and grow stronger. Greek yogurt will provide protein to your hair, apple cider vinegar will cleanse it, and honey will help seal moisture. This hair mask is also great for hair fall.

Ingredients:
  1 cup yogurt
  2 tbsp apple cider vinegar
  1 tbsp honey

Directions:

1) Combine all ingredients to make your yogurt hair mask.

2) Apply to your hair from roots to tips and leave for 15 minutes to dry.

3) Rinse well with water and shampoo and condition as usual.

Rice Water and Avocado Hair Mask for Healthier Curls

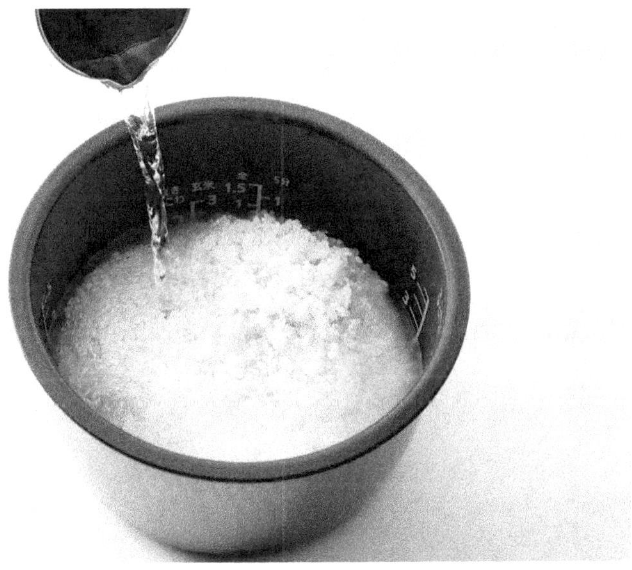

Inositol is a component of rice water that can permeate the hair and repair any damage. Avocado also has a high amount of vitamin B-complex, which aids hair development and is highly moisturizing. This homemade hair mask will help your curls reclaim their vitality and definition.

Ingredients:

   1 cup of rice

   2 cups of water

   ½ avocado

Directions:

1) Mash half an avocado to make this hair mask, and soak 1 cup of rice in 2 cups of water.

2) Sieve the mixture to remove the rice grains from the water.

3) Toss in the avocado mash with the rice water.

4) Apply it to your hair and scalp.

5) Allow 20 to 25 minutes to sit on your hair before washing it with warm water and a light shampoo.

Banana and Avocado Hair Mask For Limp and Dry Hair

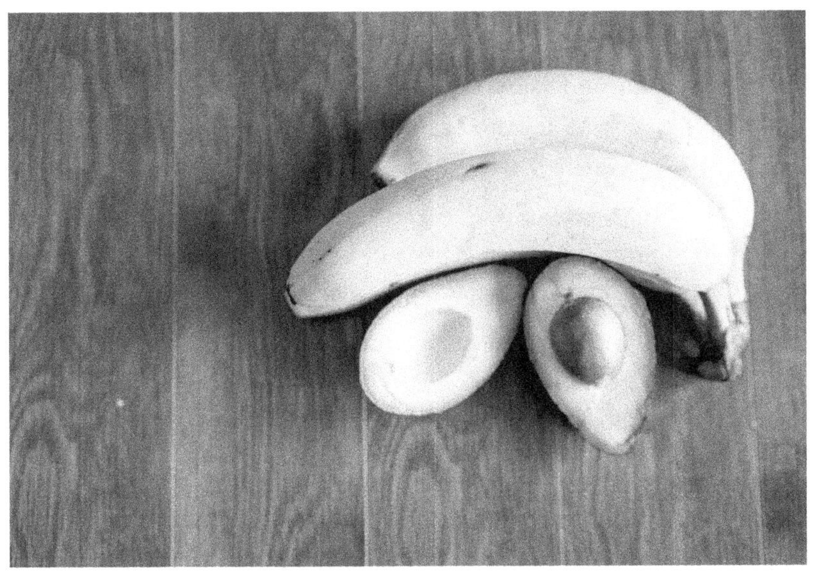

Curly hair is notorious for being incredibly dry and frizzy. Furthermore, heat style, sun damage, and regular exposure to the elements aggravate by leaving it dull and brittle, robbing it of its original texture. Quench your thirsty hair with this ultra-moisturizing and nourishing hair mask that will strengthen your strands while adding bounce and gloss to your natural curl.

Ingredients:

   1 banana

   ½ avocado

   3 tsp mayo

   2 tsp virgin coconut oil

   2 tsp castor oil

   1 egg (optional)

Directions:

1) mash the banana and avocado together in a large mixing bowl. Combine the mayonnaise, coconut oil, castor oil, and egg.

2) Mix till you get a smooth paste.

3) Apply generously to damp, shampooed hair in sections, focusing on each part from root to tip.

3) Put on the shower cap and let your hair absorb the mask for about an hour after applying it to your entire hair.

4) Rinse well with cold water.

Baking Soda Hair Mask for Product Buildup

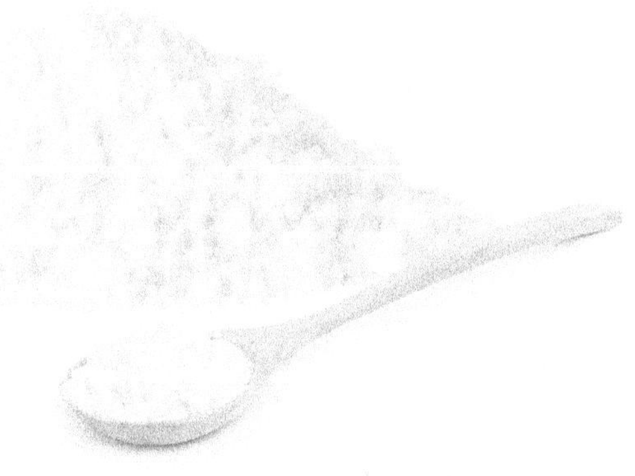

It's easy to build up layers of residue from hair care and styling products, especially for curly hair. Buildup can cause greasy-looking and feeling strands, dullness, and even dandruff-like flakes. With this baking soda hair mask, you can eliminate excess oil and buildup.

Ingredients:
   half a cup of shampoo
   1-2 tbsp baking soda

Directions:
   1) Combine shampoo and baking soda in a mixing bowl, stir well, and apply to damp hair.
   2) Massage the mixture into your scalp gently and let it stay for a few minutes before thoroughly washing.

Coconut Cream, Cocoa Powder, and Cinnamon for Thinning Hair

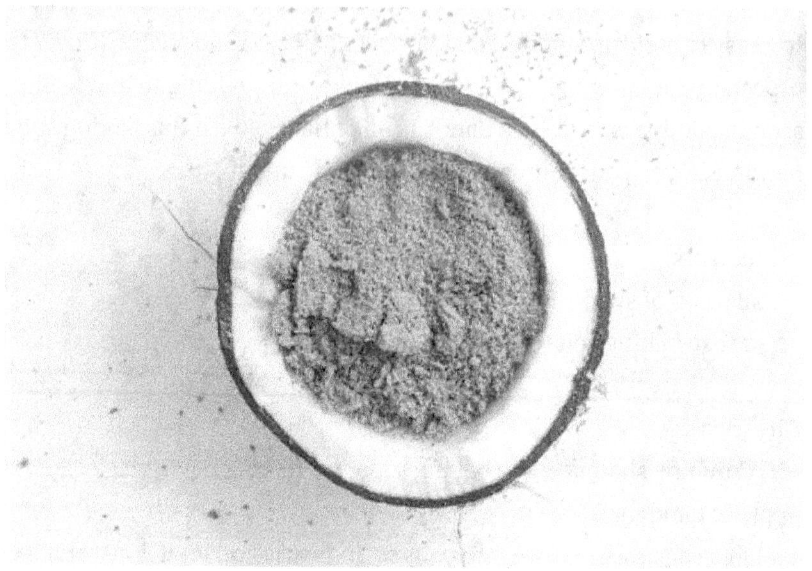

The theobromine in the cocoa powder boosts growth by boosting blood flow. Cinnamon increases circulation around hair follicles. Both of these contribute to this mask's ability to promote thickness.

Ingredients:

    5 ounces of coconut cream/coconut milk
    ½ cup of no-sugar-added cocoa powder
    ¾ tablespoon of powdered cinnamon

Directions:

1. Mash the ripe avocado until it's nice and creamy.
2. Mix in the honey.
3. Apply this creamy mix to your hair, covering it from roots to tips.
4. Leave it on for about 20-30 minutes.
5. Rinse it out thoroughly with warm water.

Avocado and Honey Mask:

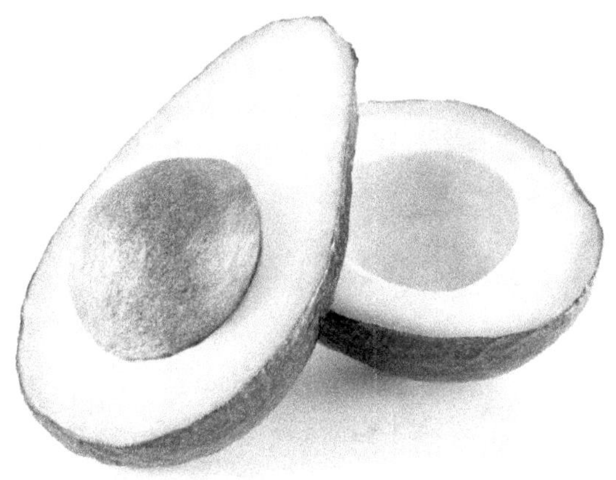

Imagine your hair getting a yummy snack. That's what an avocado and honey mask does.

Ingredients:

A ripe avocado

Honey (about 2 tablespoons)

Directions:

1. Mash the ripe avocado until it's nice and creamy.

2. Mix in the honey.

3. Apply this creamy mix to your hair, covering it from roots to tips.

4. Leave it on for about 20-30 minutes.

5. Rinse it out thoroughly with warm water.

Why It's Awesome:

Avocado contains healthy fats and vitamins that hydrate and strengthen your hair. Honey is a natural humectant, which means it locks in moisture.

Aloe Vera as a Natural Hair Gel

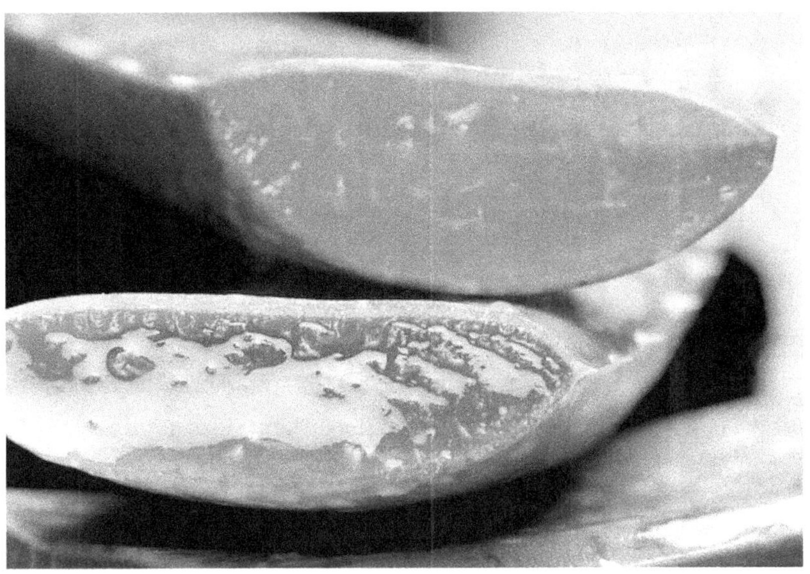

Aloe vera isn't just for soothing sunburns; it can also be a fantastic hair gel alternative.

Ingredients:

Aloe vera gel: extract it from an aloe vera leaf or buy it pre-made. Aloe vera is super hydrating and helps reduce frizz. It's gentle on your hair and scalp, making it a natural choice for curly hair.

Directions:

1. Take a small amount of aloe vera gel in your hands.
2. Rub your hands together to warm it up a bit.
3. Apply it to your hair like you would with regular hair gel.
4. Style your curls as desired.

These DIY treatments and solutions are like little homemade miracles for your curls. They're simple, fun to make, and can give your hair the love and care it deserves. So, get ready to have fabulous, healthy curls!

3.4 Methods for applying hair styling products

1. Squish-to-Condish Method: After applying the conditioner, you scrunch your hair soaked in water to help the product distribute evenly and encourage curl formation. Then, rinse gently.
2. Plopping: After showering, wrap your wet hair in a microfiber towel or a cotton T-shirt, allowing it to absorb excess water and encourage curl formation.
3. The LCO, LOCG, and LOCJ methods are variations of the popular LOC method, used by people with curly and natural hair to help lock in moisture and keep their hair hydrated and defined. These methods involve layering specific products to maximize moisture retention. Let's break down each method:

1. LCO Method:

Note: The L in this method can be a leave-in conditioner or liquid (water).

L - Leave-In Conditioner: Start with a leave-in conditioner to give your hair initial moisture. Apply it evenly throughout your hair, focusing on the ends.

C - Cream: Next, apply a creamy product like curl-defining or styling cream. This step helps seal the moisture from the leave-in conditioner and adds definition to your curls. Distribute the cream evenly through your hair.

O - Oil: Finish with an oil-based product such as hair oil or serum. The oil helps lock in the moisture the leave-in conditioner and cream provide, creating a protective barrier. It also adds shine to your curls.

The LCO method benefits people with thicker or coarser hair because it emphasizes the sealing properties of the cream and oil.

2. LOCG Method:

L - Leave-In Conditioner: As in the LCO method, begin with a leave-in conditioner to hydrate your curls.

O - Oil: Apply an oil-based product after the leave-in conditioner. This step locks in the moisture from the conditioner and creates a barrier against humidity.

C - Cream: Follow up with a curl-defining or styling cream to further seal in the moisture. The cream helps with curl definition and control.

G - Gel: Finish with gel to provide hold and control frizz. The gel locks in the moisture from the previous steps and helps maintain your curls' shape.

The LOCG method is often chosen by individuals who live in humid climates or have hair that is prone to frizz. The gel step offers extra frizz control and curl definition.

3. LOCJ Method:

L - Leave-In Conditioner: To hydrate your curls, begin with a leave-in conditioner.

O - Oil: Apply an oil-based product after the leave-in conditioner to seal in the moisture.

C - Cream: Add a curl-defining or styling cream to add definition.

J - Jelly or Jelly-like Product: Finish with a jelly or jelly-like styling product. These products help hold curls in place and offer extra definition.

The LOCJ method is a variation that includes a jelly or jelly-like product as the final step to provide enhanced hold and curl definition.

These methods are about finding the right combination of products and order that works best for your hair type and personal preferences. Experimenting with different products and techniques can help you achieve the moisture, definition, and style desired for your curly hair.

Common Techniques for Applying Product:

- Praying hands method: a technique for smoothing styling product over curly hair to prevent frizz.
- Rack and Shake: a technique that applies products by sectioning the hair and raking styling products from roots to ends. Holding hair at the ends and gently shake your hair to form natural curls.
- Combing products: A technique that uses a wide-tooth comb to apply styling products. Section the hair, apply your product, and follow with a comb to ensure product distribution.

3.5 Gels vs. Creams: Which to Choose?

Choosing between gels and creams is an essential decision regarding curly hair products. Here's a breakdown to help you decide which one might be the better fit for your curls:

Gels:

Hold and Definition: Gels are known for their stronghold and ability to define curls, making them a great choice to maintain your curl pattern and keep frizz at bay.

Lightweight: They are lightweight and won't weigh down your curls.

Wet Look: Gels can give your curls a damp or shiny appearance, which some people love for a sleek, polished look.

Humidity Control: Gels are excellent at combating humidity and preventing frizz, making them ideal for those in humid climates.

Creams:

Hydration: Creams are moisturizing and can give your curls the hydration they need, making them an excellent choice for drier hair types.

Softer Hold: They typically offer a softer hold than gels, which can be great for those who prefer a more natural or bouncy look.

Anti-Frizz: Creams often have anti-frizz properties, helping to keep your curls smooth and well-behaved.

Volume: If you're looking for volume and fullness, creams can help add body to your curls.

How to Choose:

Hair Type: Consider your hair type and needs. Creams work better for you if you have fine or loose curls. If you have coarser or tighter curls, gels may be more effective.

Desired Look: Think about the style you want to achieve. If you prefer defined, sleek curls, go for a gel. Opt for a cream if you want a softer, more natural look. Use a cream and gel or jelly to seal and hold your style.

Climate: Your local climate can play a role. A gel might be your best defense against frizz if you live in a humid area. Ultimately, there's no one-size-fits-all answer, and you can even experiment with gels and creams to find what combination works best for your curls.

3.6 Avoiding Harmful Ingredients: How to Avoid Them and Which Ingredients to Avoid

It's crucial to avoid harmful ingredients in some hair products. Here are some tips on how to avoid them and a list of common ingredients to watch out for.

How to Avoid Harmful Ingredients:

1. Read Labels: Always read the ingredient labels on hair products before purchasing. Look for products that are free of harmful additives.
2. Research Brands: Research and choose brands that prioritize natural and safe ingredients.
3. Use Apps/Websites: Consider using apps and websites that help you analyze product ingredients for safety (e.g., "Think Dirty" or "EWG's Skin Deep").

Ingredients to Avoid in Curly Hair Products:

1. Sulfates can be harsh and dry. Look for sodium lauryl sulfate (SLS)

and ammonium lauryl sulfate (ALS).

2. Silicones: Some silicones can cause buildup and prevent moisture from penetrating your hair. Common ones include dimethicone and cyclomethicone.

3. Parabens: These are preservatives that can be potentially harmful. Look for ingredients like methylparaben and propylparaben.

4. Alcohols: Some alcohols can dry your curls. Avoid products with ingredients like denatured alcohol and isopropyl alcohol.

5. Mineral Oil and Petrolatum: These can create a barrier that may block moisture absorption.

6. Artificial Fragrances: Synthetic fragrances can cause irritation. Opt for products with natural fragrances or none at all.

7. Phthalates: These are often hidden under "fragrance" in ingredient lists and can have adverse health effects.

By being vigilant about product ingredients and choosing those free from harmful substances, you can help your curly hair stay healthy, hydrated, and beautiful.

Protective Styles for Curl Preservation

Here are five easy protective styles suitable for anyone:

1. Pineapple Updo: Gather your curls into a high, loose ponytail on your head, secured with a scrunchie or silk scarf to preserve curls while sleeping

2. Braided Crown: Create a loose braid around the crown of your head, leaving the rest of your curls free. It protects your hair and adds a stylish touch.

3. Low Bun: Gather your curls into a low bun secured with a hair-friendly scrunchie, keeping them safe and neat.

4. Twists or Mini-Braids: Divide your hair into small sections and twist or braid each section. This style protects your curls and adds texture when you take them down.

5. Headscarf Wrap: Tie a colorful scarf around your head, covering your curls completely to protect them from friction and environmental factors.

4

Chapter 4: Curly Hair Challenges

4.1 Combatting Frizz and Humidity for Different Hair Types

Imagine Frizz as a wild-haired rebel who won't obey the rules. And guess what? Humidity (moisture in the air) can make them even naughtier! But fear not; different hair types have their own secret weapons to tame the frizz.

For Loose Curls (Type 2):

Product Recommendations:

- Shea Moisture Coconut & Hibiscus Curl Enhancing Smoothie
- Moroccanoil Curl Defining Cream
- Camille Rose Naturals Curlaide Moisture Butter

For Tight Curls (Type 3):

Product Recommendations:

- Cantu Shea Butter for Natural Hair Moisturizing Curl Activator Cream
- Ouidad Advanced Climate Control Heat & Humidity Gel
- Mielle Organics Pomegranate & Honey Curl Smoothie
- For Coily Curls (Type 4):

Product Recommendations:

- Shea Moisture Jamaican Black Castor Oil Strengthen & Restore Leave-In Conditioner
- Kinky-Curly Original Curling Custard Natural Styling Gel
- Aunt Jackie's Curl La La Defining Curl Custard
- 4.2 Addressing Dryness and Breakage for Different Hair Types

For Loose Curls (Type 2):

Product Recommendations:

- OGX Moroccan Argan Oil Shampoo & Conditioner
- Bumble and Bumble Hairdresser's Invisible Oil Primer
- Not Your Mother's Naturals Tahitian Gardenia Flower & Mango Butter Curl Defining Detangler

For Tight Curls (Type 3):

Product Recommendations:

- As I Am Coconut CoWash Cleansing Conditioner
- Mielle Organics Babassu Oil & Mint Deep Conditioner
- Curls Blueberry Bliss Reparative Hair Mask

For Coily Curls (Type 4):

Product Recommendations:

- Shea Moisture Raw Shea Butter Moisture Retention Shampoo & Restorative Conditioner
- Aunt Jackie's Knot On My Watch Instant Detangling Therapy
- Taliah Waajid Protective Styles Bamboo, Biotin & Basil Nourishing Hair & Scalp Serum

4.3 Handling Curl Variations (Different Curls on One Head)

Sometimes, your curls are like a diverse group of friends, each with their own style. That's the fun of it! Here's how to keep everyone happy:

Your Strategy: Use a particular curl product that suits the tighter curls; go with something light and breezy for the looser ones.

Product Recommendations:

- For tighter curls: Camille Rose Naturals Curl Maker.
- For looser curls, OGX Quenching Coconut Curls Curling Butter Leave-In or Cantu Moisturizing Curl Activator Cream.
- Embracing your unique curls is all about finding the right curly hair heroes and having fun. So, let your curls be the stars they were born to be!

Tips for Managing Your Curls:

1. Moisture is Key: Curly hair tends to be drier than straight hair, so invest in a good conditioner and use it regularly.

2. Avoid Heat: Heat-styling tools like straighteners can damage your curls. Embrace your natural texture or use heat sparingly and with heat-protectant products.

3. Detangle Carefully: Use a wide-toothed comb or your fingers to detangle your hair when wet and full of conditioner to prevent breakage. Detangle by starting with the ends and working up a wide-toothed comb.

4. Find the Right Products: Experiment with different products like curl enhancers, gels, or creams to find what works best for your curls.

5. Protect at Night: Consider using a satin or silk pillowcase to prevent friction and frizz. You can also use a silk or satin bonnet.

6. Regular Trims: Get regular trims to keep your curls looking fresh and healthy.

Remember, there's no one-size-fits-all approach to curly hair care. What works best for you may not work for someone else, so be patient and embrace your unique curls. With a bit of care and the right products, you can confidently rock those curls!

5

Chapter 5: Tips for Specific Curl Types

5.1 Wavy Hair (Type 2A, 2B, 2C)

Wavy hair is like the beautiful ocean waves – it's not straight, but not super curly, either. Here are some tips and products to help wavy-haired folks:

Common Problems:

- Wavies often deal with frizz, especially in humid weather.
- Sometimes, waves can look limp and lack definition.

Styling Products:

- Frizz Control Serum: Look for a lightweight frizz control serum to smooth those frizzies. A product like John Frieda Frizz Ease Extra Strength Serum works well.
- Wave-Enhancing Spray: Try a wave-enhancing spray, such as Bumble and Bumble Surf Spray, to give your waves that beachy, textured look.

- Lightweight Mousse: A light mousse-like TRESemmé TRES Two Extra Hold Hair Mousse can add volume and hold without weighing down your waves.

DIY Masks/Treatments:

Coconut Oil Mask: This helps with hydration and adds shine.

- Warm up some coconut oil.
- Apply it to your hair.
- Leave it on for about 30 minutes.

Honey and Yogurt Mask: It's a natural way to boost moisture and definition.

- Mix honey and plain yogurt and apply to your hair.
- Let it sit for 20-30 minutes.
- Wash hair and style as usual.

5.2 Curly Hair (Type 3A, 3B, 3C)

Curly hair is like a beautiful spiral dance! Here are some tips and products to help those with curly hair:

Common Problems:

- Curly hair can be prone to frizz, especially in humidity.
- Maintaining curl definition and bounce can be a challenge.
- Hair Products:

Styling Products:

- Curl-Defining Cream: Look for a curl-defining cream like Shea Moisture Coconut & Hibiscus Curl Enhancing Smoothie to keep those curls looking their best.
- Anti-Frizz Serum: An anti-frizz serum, such as Garnier Fructis Sleek & Shine Anti-Frizz Serum, can help keep your curls smooth and shiny.
- Leave-In Conditioner: A good leave-in conditioner like Ouidad Moisture.

DIY Masks/Treatments: This DIY mask adds moisture and shine.

Banana and Olive Oil Mask:

- Blend a ripe banana with olive oil.
- Apply it to your hair.
- Leave it on for 20-30 minutes.

Apple Cider Vinegar Rinse: It helps with detangling and adds shine.

- Mix apple cider vinegar with water (about 1:3 ratio).
- Use it as a final rinse after shampooing and conditioning.

5.3 Coily Hair (Type 4A, 4B, 4C)

Coily hair is all about those tight, beautiful coils! Here are some tips and products to help coily-haired individuals:

Common Problems:

- Coily hair often craves moisture to prevent dryness and breakage.
- Taming frizz and maintaining curl definition are key challenges.
- Hair Products:

Styling Products:

Hydrating Leave-In Conditioner: A hydrating leave-in conditioner like Cantu Shea Butter Leave-In Conditioning Repair Cream can be a lifesaver for coily hair.

Curl-Defining Gel: A curl-defining gel such as Kinky-Curly Original Curling Custard can help you achieve defined coils.

Hair Oil: A natural hair oil like Jamaican Black Castor Oil can provide extra moisture and help seal the hair cuticle.

DIY Masks/Treatments: This deep treatment helps with moisture and curl definition.

Shea Butter and Aloe Vera Mask:

- Mix shea butter with aloe vera gel.
- Apply to your hair.
- Leave it on for 30-45 minutes.

Avocado and Coconut Oil Mask: It's a nourishing treat for your coils, adding moisture and shine.

- Blend avocado with coconut oil and apply to your hair,
- Leave it on for 30 minutes.
- Then rinse your hair thoroughly and style as usual. (You can use

shampoo or conditioner to help rinse your hair thoroughly.)

These tips, products, and DIY treatments are like secret weapons tailored to your curl type, helping you keep your hair healthy, happy, and fabulous!

6

Chapter 6: Daily and Nightly Routines

6.1 Morning Refresh for Vibrant Curls

Imagine waking up to curls full of life and bounce! That's what the morning refresh is all about. Here's how it works for different curly hair types:

For Wavy Hair (Type 2A, 2B, 2C):

Morning Routine: Spritz your hair with a water and conditioner mix (about 1 part conditioner to 3 parts water) to revive your waves. Scrunch your hair gently to enhance the curls.

For Curly Hair (Type 3A, 3B, 3C):

Morning Routine: Use a spray bottle filled with water and a little leave-in conditioner to dampen your curls. Then, scrunch your hair upward to reshape those beautiful curls.

For Coily Hair (Type 4A, 4B, 4C):

Morning Routine: Moisten your hair with water and a leave-in conditioner. Next, use your fingers to re-form your coils. You can even gently shape your hair with a satin or silk scarf.

6.2 Nighttime Routine to Preserve Curls

Your curls need their beauty sleep, too! Here's how to keep them in tip-top shape overnight:

For Wavy Hair (Type 2A, 2B, 2C):

Nighttime Routine: Sleep on a satin or silk pillowcase to reduce friction and prevent frizz. You can also loosely twist your hair into a loose bun on your head and secure it with a scrunchie.

For Curly Hair (Type 3A, 3B, 3C):

Nighttime Routine: Pineapple your curls into a high, loose ponytail on your head. Cover it with a satin or silk scarf or bonnet to protect your curls while you sleep. I prefer a satin or silk pillowcase. The choice is yours!

For Coily Hair (Type 4A, 4B, 4C):

Nighttime Routine: Twist or braid your hair gently into sections before bed. Cover it with a satin or silk bonnet or scarf. It preserves your coils and minimizes tangling.

These daily and nightly routines are like your curly hair's best friend, helping you keep those curls looking fresh and fabulous all day and night.

7

Chapter 7: Lifestyle and Curly Hair

7.1 Diet and Nutrition for Healthy Curls

Taking care of your curls isn't just about what you put on your hair; it's also about what you put in your body. Your diet and nutrition play a significant role in the health of your curls.

Water: Drinking enough water keeps your hair hydrated from the inside out. Aim for about eight glasses a day.

Protein: Hair is made of protein, so including lean meats, fish, eggs, and beans in your diet can help maintain strong, healthy curls.

Omega-3 Fatty Acids: These are found in foods like salmon, walnuts, and flaxseeds. They help keep your hair shiny and moisturized.

Vitamins and Minerals: Nutrients like vitamins A, C, E, and biotin, as well as minerals like zinc and iron, are essential for hair health. You can find these in a balanced diet with plenty of fruits and vegetables.

7.2 Exercise and Sweat Management

Exercise is excellent for your overall health but can sometimes lead to sweaty situations for your curls. Here's how to manage it:

Sweatbands: Wearing a sweatband or headband can help keep sweat away from your hairline during workouts.

Protective Styles: Consider putting your hair in a protective style like braids or a bun while exercising to minimize friction and sweat absorption.

Dry Shampoo: After your workout, you can use dry shampoo to refresh your roots and absorb excess sweat.

7.3 Swimming and Chlorine Protection

Swimming can be fun, but chlorine in pools can be harsh on your curls. Here's how to protect them:

Pre-Swim Treatment: Wet your hair with fresh water before entering the pool. It helps your hair absorb less chlorine.

Swim Cap: Consider wearing a swim cap to create a barrier between your curls and the pool water.

After swimming, rinse your hair thoroughly with fresh water to remove chlorine, and then follow up with a deep conditioner.

Clarifying Shampoo: Use a clarifying shampoo occasionally to remove any chlorine buildup.

Taking care of your curls isn't just about hair products; it's also about making choices in your daily life, like staying hydrated, protecting your hair during exercise, and taking precautions when swimming. These lifestyle choices can help you maintain healthy and beautiful curls.

8

Conclusion

You've learned that your curls are like no one else's—each twist and turn is uniquely yours. And guess what? That's something to celebrate! Your curls are a part of your story your identity, and are absolutely fabulous.

Throughout this journey, you've discovered the science behind those locks, the secret ingredients to look for (and avoid!) in your products, and even some cool DIY tricks. You've tamed frizz, battled dryness, and learned to make your curls pop.

But remember, embracing your natural curls isn't just about the right products or routines; it's about self-love and confidence. Your curls are your crown, your superpower! They're a statement of who you are and should be celebrated, not hidden away.

So, wear your curls with pride, let them bounce, and don't be afraid to show them off. It's your time to shine, curl by curl, wave by wave. Embrace the natural beauty that is uniquely and wonderfully you.

Now, go out there and rock those curls because the world deserves to see the fantastic, curly-haired person you are!

52

9

Suggested Online Resources

YouTube, Instagram Tik-Tok, Facebook

- Manes by Mell: She offers super helpful tips. She is a licensed professional hair stylist. She has been one of my go-to hair gurus since I began my curly hair journey.
- Bianca Renee Today: She offers excellent tips and reviews products for all budgets, and I love her shopping trips to the local shopping center.
- Curly Proverbs, founded by Farida Sharma as a YouTube channel, offers excellent DIY hair care recipes; she has also created her product line.

Other Recommended Hair Care Products:

- Mielle
- Not Your Mothers
- Dippity Do Curls Gelee
- Innersence

Note: I only speak for myself and my experiences using these products and viewing the mentioned channels. I have not been paid to recommend these products or online media.

54

10

Reference

Best Hair Dryer For Curly Hair: Frizz-Free And Care-Free 2023. https://allwomenhairstyles.com/best-hair-dryer-for-curly-hair/

Hair Porosity 101 with the Ultimate Care and Styling Tips. https://therighthairstyles.com/hair-porosity?utm_medium=cpc&utm_campaign=link

Best Shampoo For Hair Fall In 2023 - Expert Recommended - Kama Ayurveda. https://www.kamaayurveda.in/blog/best-shampoo-for-hair-fall

Best Shampoo For Hair Fall In 2023 - Expert Recommended - Kama Ayurveda. https://www.kamaayurveda.in/blog/best-shampoo-for-hair-fall

How Often Should You Wash Permed Hair? - Lauren+Vanessa. https://laurenandvanessa.com/how-often-should-you-wash-permed-hair/

Best Way To Prevent Frizz For Afro Hair Types | Nylah's Naturals. https://www.nylahsnaturals.com/blogs/news/best-way-to-prevent -frizz-for-afro-hair-types

Cantu Shea Butter For Natural Hair Sulfate-Free Cleansing Cream Shampoo – Omii Hair. https://omiihair.com/collections/cantu/pro ducts/cantu-shea-butter-for-natural-hair-sulfate-free-cleansing- cream-shampoo

"The Benefits of Aloe Vera for Curly Hair." Hairfood.Com, 2 Jan. 2023, hairfood.com/en-us/our-blogs/benefits-of-aloe-vera-curly-hair/

Is Root To End Good For Your Hair? Debunking The Myths And Facts - Coloringfolder.com. https://coloringfolder.com/is-root-to-end-go od-for-your-hair-debunking-the-myths-and-facts/

6 DIY Hair Masks for Curly Hair That Are Sure To Work – Burlybands. https://burlybands.com/blogs/news/6-diy-hair-masks-for-curly- hair-that-are-sure-to-work

Shea Moisture Jamaican Black Castor Oil Strengthen & Restore Leave- .... https://123hair.nl/en/shea-moisture-jamaican-black-castor-oil -strengthen-restore-leave-in-conditioner-312-gr.html

The Best Products Like DevaCurl That Protect Your Locks. https://chic pursuit.com/products-like-devacurl/

SHEA MOISTURE RAW SHEA BUTTER MOISTURE RETENTION SHAM- POO 13oz. https://bswbeautyca.com/products/shea-moisture-raw- shea-butter-moisture-retention-shampoo

How do I get the prettiest curls - Home Automation Technology. http://homeautotechs.com/How-do-I-get-the-prettiest-curls/

How To Grow African American Hair Fast? | Straightener Lab. https://www.straightenerlab.com/how-to-grow-african-american-hair-fast/

Maintaining Healthy, Growing Hair - What You Need To Know – SuperFoodLx. https://superfoodlx.com/blogs/news/expert-tips-for-maintaining-healthy-growing-hair

Boosting NAD+ Production Naturally – Avior Nutritionals - NADIA. https://nadiaskin.com/blogs/nadia/boosting-nad-production-naturally

Clever Life Hacks Every Girl Should Know. https://medical-news.org/clever-life-hacks-every-girl-should-know/47108/19/

www.ingramcontent.com/pod-product-compliance
Lightning Source LLC
Chambersburg PA
CBHW070723260726
48660CB00007B/2699